A Checklist for Dad

Written by Dr Tricia L. Larose

Illustrated by Gwen Le Rest

Edited by Beth Cox

Designed by Gary Peters, Fossil Design

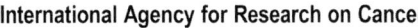
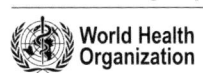
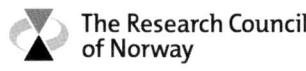
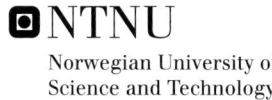

Published by the International Agency for Research on Cancer,
150 cours Albert Thomas, 69372 Lyon Cedex 08, France

© International Agency for Research on Cancer, 2020

Distributed by: WHO Press, World Health Organization, 20 Avenue Appia, 1211 Geneva 27, Switzerland
(tel: +41 22 791 3264; fax: +41 22 791 4857; email: bookorders@who.int).

Publications of the World Health Organization enjoy copyright protection in accordance with the provisions of Protocol 2 of the Universal Copyright Convention. All rights reserved.

The designations employed and the presentation of the material in this publication do not imply the expression of any opinion whatsoever on the part of the Secretariat of the World Health Organization concerning the legal status of any country, territory, city, or area or of its authorities or concerning the delimitation of its frontiers or boundaries.

The mention of specific companies or of certain manufacturers' products does not imply that they are endorsed or recommended by the World Health Organization in preference to others of a similar nature that are not mentioned. Errors and omissions excepted, the names of proprietary products are distinguished by initial capital letters.

The authors alone are responsible for the views expressed in this publication.

The International Agency for Research on Cancer welcomes requests for permission to reproduce or translate its publications, in part or in full. Requests for permission to reproduce or translate IARC publications – whether for sale or for non-commercial distribution – should be addressed to the IARC Communications Group, at: publications@iarc.fr.

IARC Library Cataloguing in Publication Data

Names: Larose, Tricia L. | Le Rest, Gwen, illustrator.

Title: A Checklist for Dad / by Tricia L. Larose; illustrated by Gwen Le Rest.

Description: Lyon, France: International Agency for Research on Cancer, 2020. | Includes questions & answers.
Identifiers: ISBN 978-92-832-0449-7 (pbk)

Subjects: LCSH: Cancer – Juvenile literature | Cancer – Patient – Family relationships – Juvenile literature.
Children of cancer patient – Juvenile literature.

Classification: LCC: RC264 .L37 2020 | DDC: 616.994

This book is dedicated to children and families everywhere

100% of the proceeds from the sale of this book go to the Education and Training Group at the International Agency for Research on Cancer to support courses, fellowships, and training of cancer researchers worldwide.

Chapter One

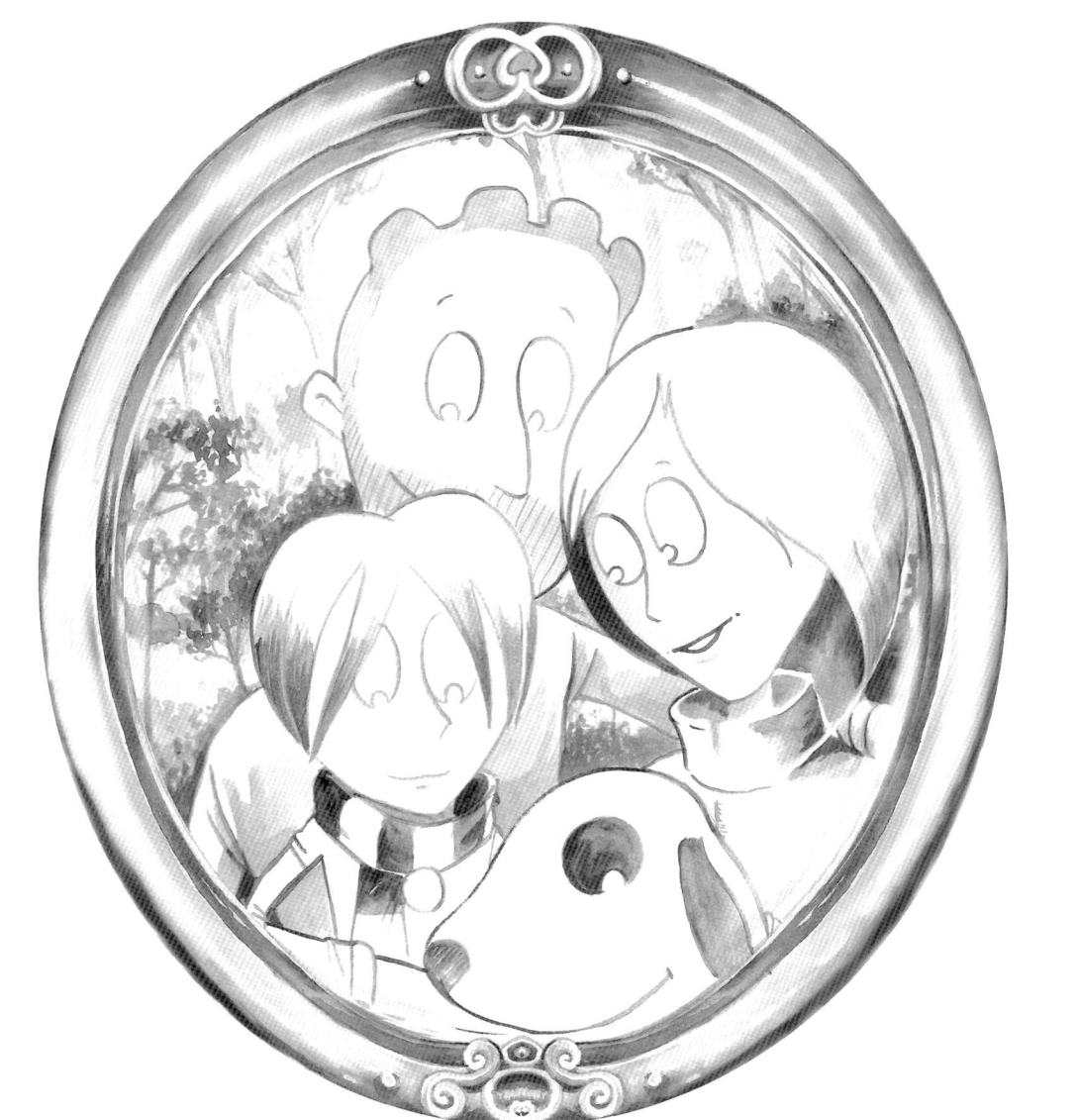

It was the middle of the night when Ella overheard her parents talking. She had woken up to go to the toilet and was surprised to see the kitchen light on. Why are Mum and Dad still awake? Ella wondered. And what are they talking about? Ella tiptoed to the toilet and back, carefully avoiding the squeaky spot on the floor. She stood quietly at the top of the stairs and squeezed her ear through the banisters.

"What did the doctor say?" asked Mum.

"I'm lucky they found it at an early stage," replied Dad. "Hopefully I won't need surgery."

"When will we know more?" asked Mum.

"I have another appointment at the hospital next week," replied Dad. "The doctors will finalise the treatment plan then."

Ella couldn't hear what Dad said next, but Mum was silent in response.

"At least my hair won't fall out," said Dad with a chuckle.

Ella was confused. She couldn't believe her ears. Dad had to go to the hospital? Dad was ill? He didn't look ill. He didn't sound ill.
Maybe I'm still asleep, thought Ella. Maybe this is all a dream.

When Ella next opened her eyes, the sun was streaming through the bedroom curtains. It was Sunday morning and the house was quiet and still.
Jasper, the family dog, was fast asleep next to Ella's bed. She was reaching down to stroke his head when she remembered hearing her parents talking.

"Dad said he had to go to the hospital," Ella whispered to Jasper, who whined in response. It doesn't make any sense, thought Ella. Mum hasn't even made him chicken noodle soup to eat. Maybe I'm wrong. Maybe I misheard.
After all, it was the middle of the night.

"Do you know what's wrong with Dad?" she asked Jasper as she slid out of bed, even though she knew he couldn't answer. "How can I find out?"
They sat together on her bedroom floor while Ella thought.

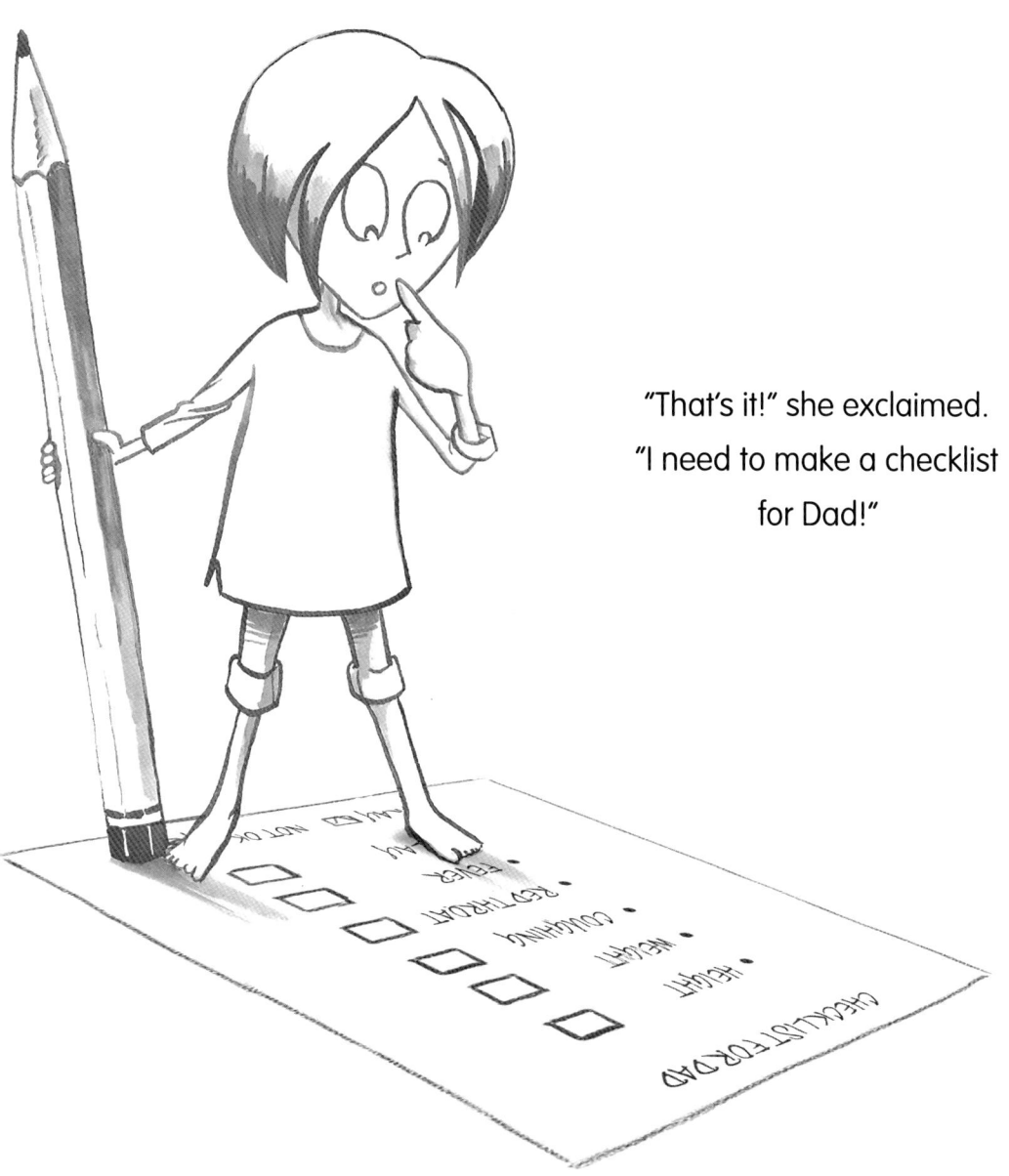

"That's it!" she exclaimed. "I need to make a checklist for Dad!"

Ella jumped up full of determination. Jasper leaped up to join her and they hurried down the stairs and straight into the kitchen to find a notebook and pen. Sitting at the table with Jasper at her feet, Ella looked down at a blank page and thought. She tried to remember the last time she was ill.

Her Mum had said her forehead was hot from a fever, and she hadn't felt like playing. Ella tapped the pen on the open notebook. Oh yes, Ella thought. The doctor looked at my throat because I had a cough. She said it was red. Ella thought back to her other visits to the family doctor. One time the doctor had measured her height and her weight.

At the top of the page Ella wrote 'Checklist for Dad'. Down the left side she wrote a list: height, weight, coughing, red throat, fever, and play. Next to each item on the list she drew a little box that she could mark off once she had checked Dad.

Just as she finished, Dad walked into the kitchen looking a little sleepy. "Good morning," he said.

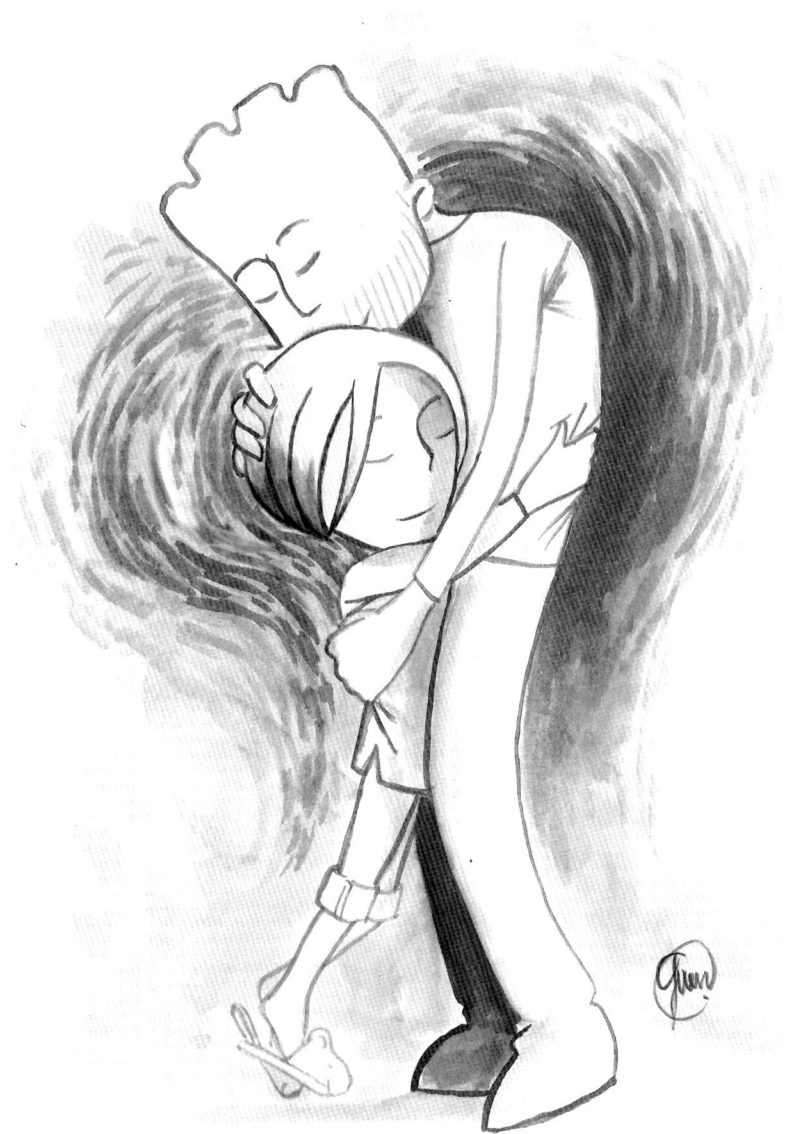

"Morning," Ella replied, quickly closing the notebook. The first two items on her list were height and weight. Easy! All I have to do is give Dad a big hug! Ella thought. She knew exactly where the top of her head should reach when she hugged Dad. She also knew that she could just touch the tips of her fingers together behind Dad's back when she gave him a hug.

Dad was leaning on the kitchen counter waiting for the kettle to boil. Ella skipped over to give him a big hug. She wrapped her arms around Dad's waist and stretched until the tips of her fingers touched together. Sure enough, Dad was just the right size. He was neither bigger nor smaller than the day before. She nuzzled her head into the spot above his belly but not quite as high as his chest. Sure enough, the top of her head was exactly where it was supposed to be. Dad was neither taller nor shorter than the day before.

"What a lovely hug," said Dad, bending over to kiss Ella's forehead.

Back at the table, Ella opened the notebook and checked off the first two boxes – one for height, and one for weight. So far, Dad was okay!

Chapter Two

Sundays were always fun. Dad would make pancakes and the family would enjoy a nice lazy breakfast together. Afterwards they would go for a long walk – even if it was raining or snowing outside. There was no school or work. Sunday was the longest, and the best, day of the week.

Ella was feeling pretty good after all the pancakes. She had almost forgotten about her checklist until she saw Mum reaching for the notebook when they were clearing the table.

"Wait!" said Ella. "I'm using that!"

Mum smiled. "Okay, dear, just remember to put it away when you're done," she said, handing the notebook back to Ella.

Ella nodded and peeked at her list. Coughing was next. She was certain that Dad had not coughed during breakfast – not even once – so she checked off the box. How can I check if Dad has a red throat or fever? Ella wondered. She stared across the table at her parents, who were reading the weekend newspapers. Aha! Ella thought. She had an idea.

CHECKLIST FOR DAD

- HEIGHT ✓
- WEIGHT ✓
- COUGHING ✓
- RED THROAT ☐
- FEVER ☐
- PLAY

OK

"Mum?" asked Ella in a quiet voice. "Can you see if my throat is red?"

Mum placed her section of the newspaper on the table and looked at Ella with a concerned frown. "Oh, sweetheart, are you feeling poorly?" asked Mum.

Ella wasn't sure what to say. She didn't want to lie. "Some kids at school were ill last week," replied Ella. "I just want to be sure I haven't caught it."
Ella stuck out her tongue and said "Ahhhhh…" just like she remembered from her visit to the doctor.

"Your throat looks fine, sweetheart," said Mum. "No need to worry."
"But what about you and Dad?" Ella asked. "We should check your throats too. Just in case."

Mum and Dad smiled at each other and then they both made funny faces as they stuck out their tongues and said "Ahhhhh."

Everyone burst out laughing, but not before Ella had a chance to look at Dad's throat. It wasn't red. Dad was still okay!

"What about a fever?" asked Ella. "We had better check if any of us have a fever." Ella's parents looked at each other again. Mum went around the table and placed the back of her hand on Ella's forehead.

"No fever," Mum confirmed.

"What about Dad?" asked Ella.

Mum placed the back of her hand on Dad's forehead. "He's fine," she said, picking up the newspaper and sitting back down.

Ella was feeling better by the moment. She held the notebook close to her chest and called for Jasper, who followed her into the other room. Ella sat quietly and looked down at her checklist. There was only one item left: play. Ella knew that if Dad really was ill, he wouldn't have the energy to play. What could she do? How could she check if Dad was up for playing?

Suddenly, Ella had an idea. She could start a tickle fight! That would be fun! Ella ran back to the kitchen and straight over to Dad.

She wiggled her fingers into his tummy. Dad laughed right away! Then Ella wiggled her fingers into Dad's armpits. It worked again – Dad was laughing!

"Come here, you little tickle monster," said Dad as he lifted Ella up into his arms and tickled her. Dad and Ella were laughing, and Jasper was jumping up and barking. They laughed and tickled each other until they were out of breath.

"Okay, you two," said Mum from the doorway. "Jasper is getting overexcited. It's time for our walk."

Dad placed Ella down on the floor and ruffled her hair. "We'd better listen to Mum," he said. "I'll make the hot chocolate to take with us."

Ella was still giggling as she walked towards the stairs. "Don't forget the oranges," she called as she ran up to get dressed. "And a treat for Jasper."

This Sunday was getting better and better with every passing moment. What a great day!

Chapter Three

The woodland park was at the edge of the city so the family usually drove there. Mum was already starting the car when Dad hollered up the stairs, "We're leaving." Jasper and Ella came running downstairs, racing out to the car.

Ella thought the park was like a magical forest. There were so many birds and squirrels in the trees, and she imagined fairies living alongside them, and elves in small mushroom houses. She loved to clamber over the huge tree roots and rocks all the way to the top of the hill.

When they finally arrived, Ella wriggled impatiently as Mum parked the car and opened the boot. Dad grabbed the rucksack and Ella raced Jasper to the footpath. Her checklist for Dad was forgotten. She was ready to be lost in the magical world of her forest. Ella started up the path with Jasper beside her. "Come on!" she yelled.

It was autumn – Ella's favourite time of year. The air smelled of pine and the footpath was covered with leaves that crunched under her feet. She rushed off ahead. "Come o-on!" she called out. Her parents were as slow as tortoises today. "You're so-o slow," she sighed, rolling her eyes in frustration.

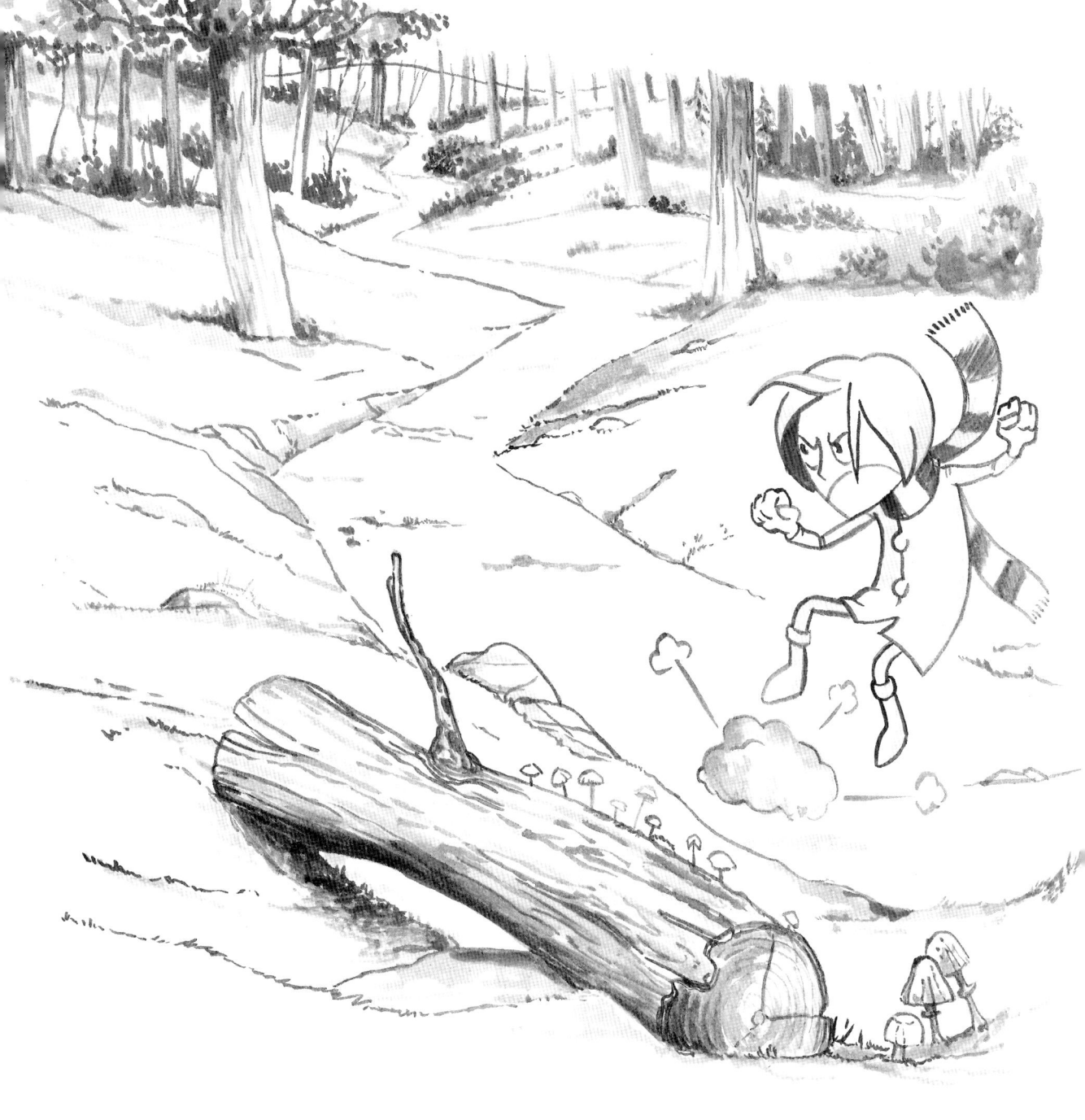

When Dad finally caught up with her, he put down the rucksack and pulled out the flask and cups.

"But Dad," complained Ella. "We're not even halfway up yet. We can't have hot chocolate until we get to the top." She was getting frustrated. The walk wasn't turning out how she'd expected. She knew they'd go home after their hot chocolate, like usual, but she wanted more time to have fun. "I don't want to go home yet!" pleaded Ella. "We've only just got here."

Mum gave Ella a hug. She pushed the loose hair from Ella's eyes and hummed softly to help soothe her. Feeling slightly better, Ella sat on an old tree stump and grudgingly accepted a cup of hot chocolate.

"Why aren't we going all the way to the top?" Ella asked grumpily. "This isn't where we normally stop."

Ella's parents looked at each other in a strange way. Ella felt uncomfortable, but she didn't know why.

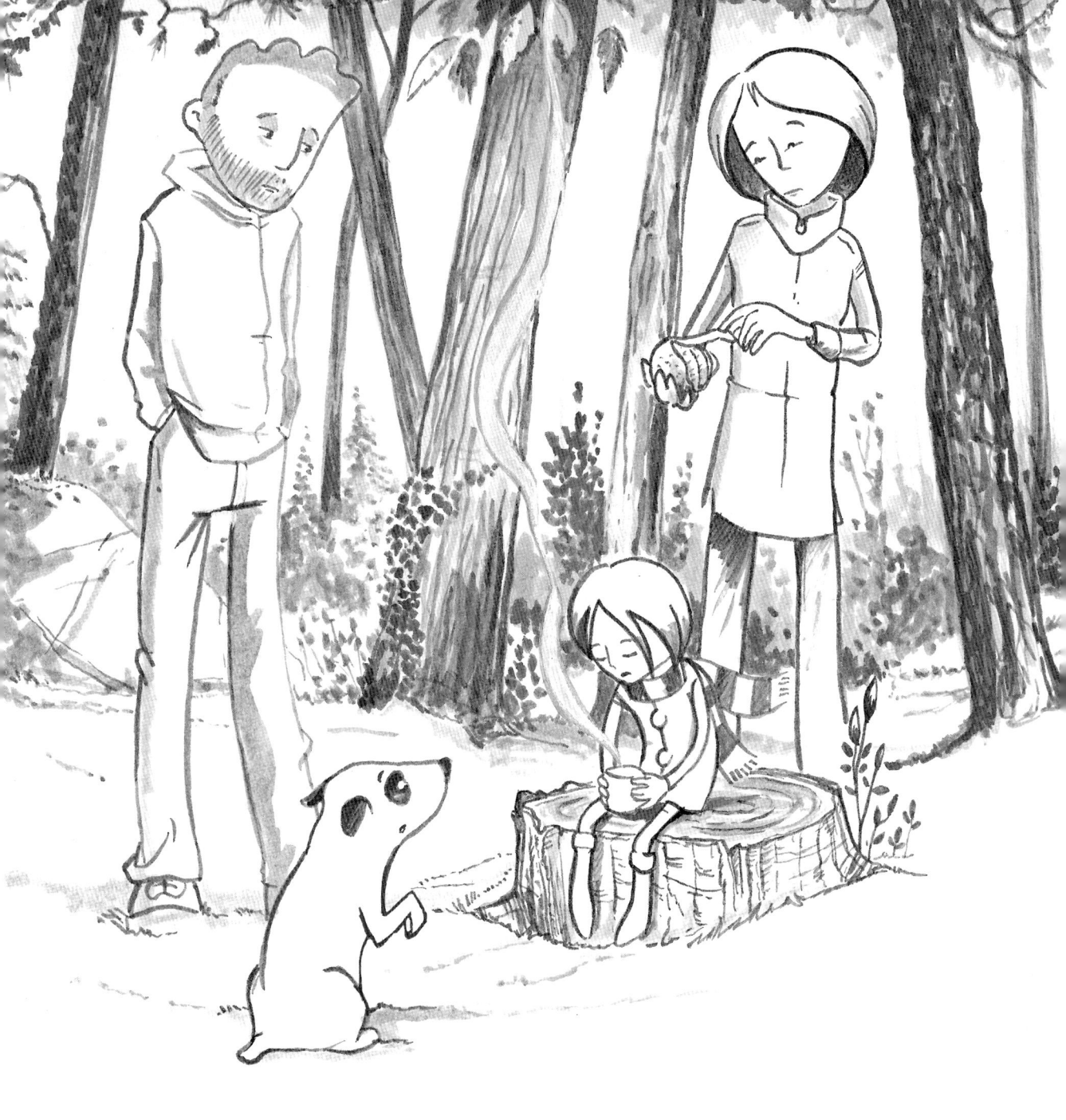

"Am I in trouble?" asked Ella.

"What makes you think that?" asked Dad.

Ella shrugged her shoulders, not sure what to say.

Mum reached into the rucksack and pulled out a juicy-looking orange. She spoke softly to Ella as she peeled it. "We found your checklist."

Ella felt like she had swallowed a stone. She had forgotten to put the notebook away. Mum must have picked it up.

"Why were you so worried about Dad?"

Ella stared at her cup and was silent for a moment.
"I heard you talking when I went to the toilet."

"Last night?" asked Mum, looking concerned.

"Last night," Ella confirmed. Her stomach was doing somersaults and her eyes were welling up.

Dad moved closer to Ella. "Oh, sweetheart," he said. "I'm so sorry you overheard us." He pulled Ella up onto his knee. "Mum and I were going to talk to you today."

Mum topped up their cups with hot chocolate.

"I'm not very well," he said. "And I've been feeling a bit more tired lately. That's why we're having a shorter walk today."

"Oh," said Ella. Her cheeks suddenly felt very warm. She looked at her dad, confused. "But you joined in the tickle fight." She didn't understand what Dad meant. "And … I checked you. You don't look ill. You don't seem ill at all."

"Indeed," agreed Dad, taking a deep breath. "I don't have a cough or a fever, and my throat isn't red. And I can still join in a tickle fight, but my body is fighting something we can't see, which makes me tired."

"What did you catch?" asked Ella.

"It's nothing I caught," replied Dad.

"Then what is it?" asked Ella. "What's wrong with you?"

Her parents looked sad and worried. When Dad finally spoke, he said, "I have cancer."

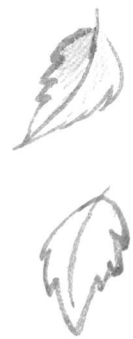
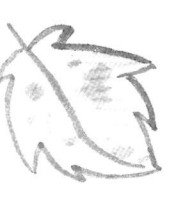
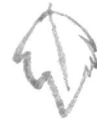

Chapter Four

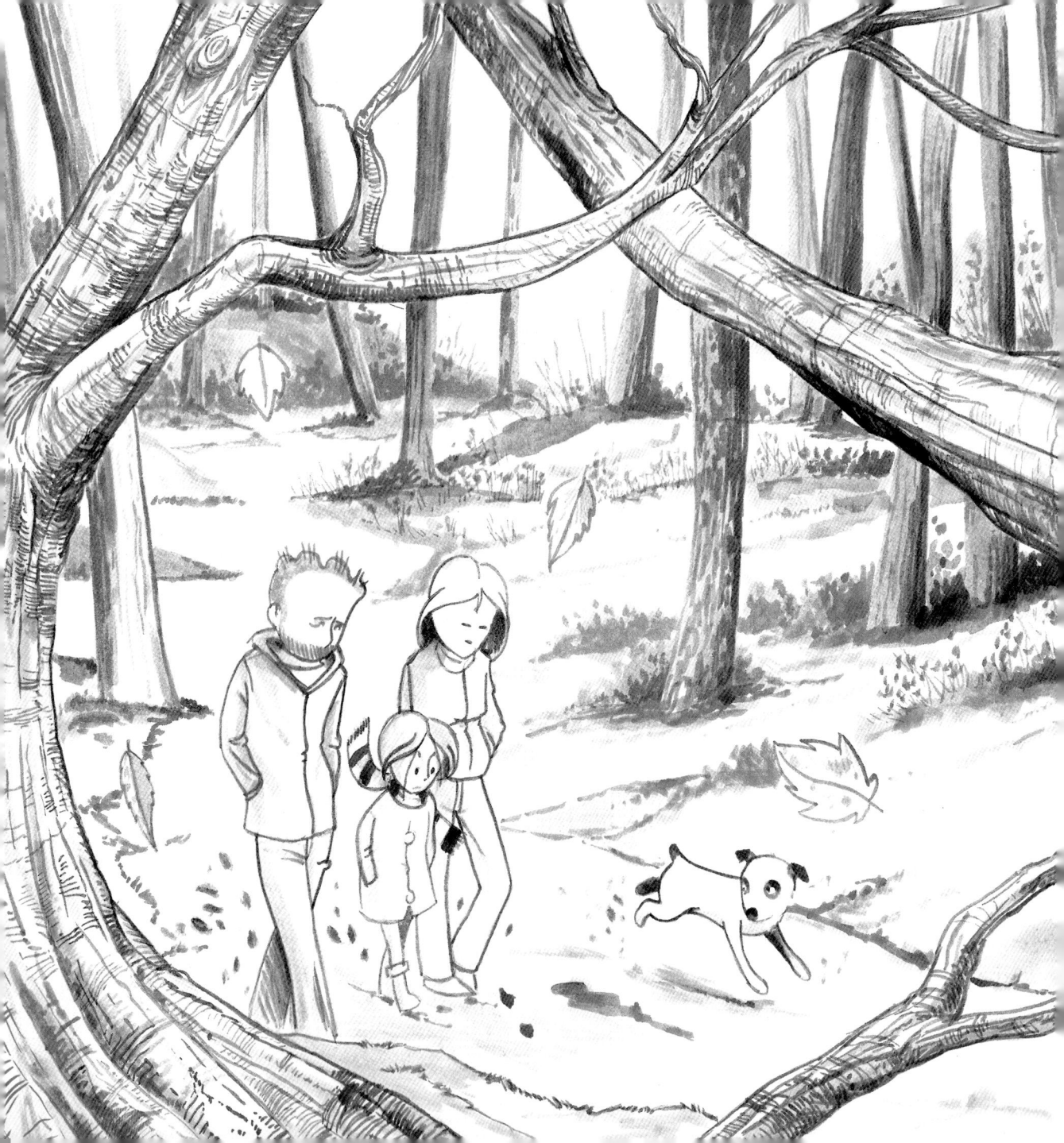

"Cancer?" asked Ella, frowning. "What's cancer?" She thought she had heard that word before, but not understanding what it meant made it sound scary.

"It's when cells in the body don't work as they should," explained Mum.

"That's right," said Dad, squeezing Ella's hand. "Cancer is quite common," Mum said, starting to pack the rucksack.

"Mum's right," added Dad, still holding Ella's hand. "Lots of different people, all over the world, get cancer. It grows in different parts of the body, and some types of cancer are more harmful than others. Some types are easier to treat than others."

"But Dad," asked Ella. "What about you?" Ella's hands were sweaty. "Can the doctors make your cancer go away?"

"I should get better," answered Dad. "I'm going to have a special treatment called radiation therapy. It'll be as if the doctor is zapping my unhealthy cells with a laser beam. Hopefully that will make the cancer go away."

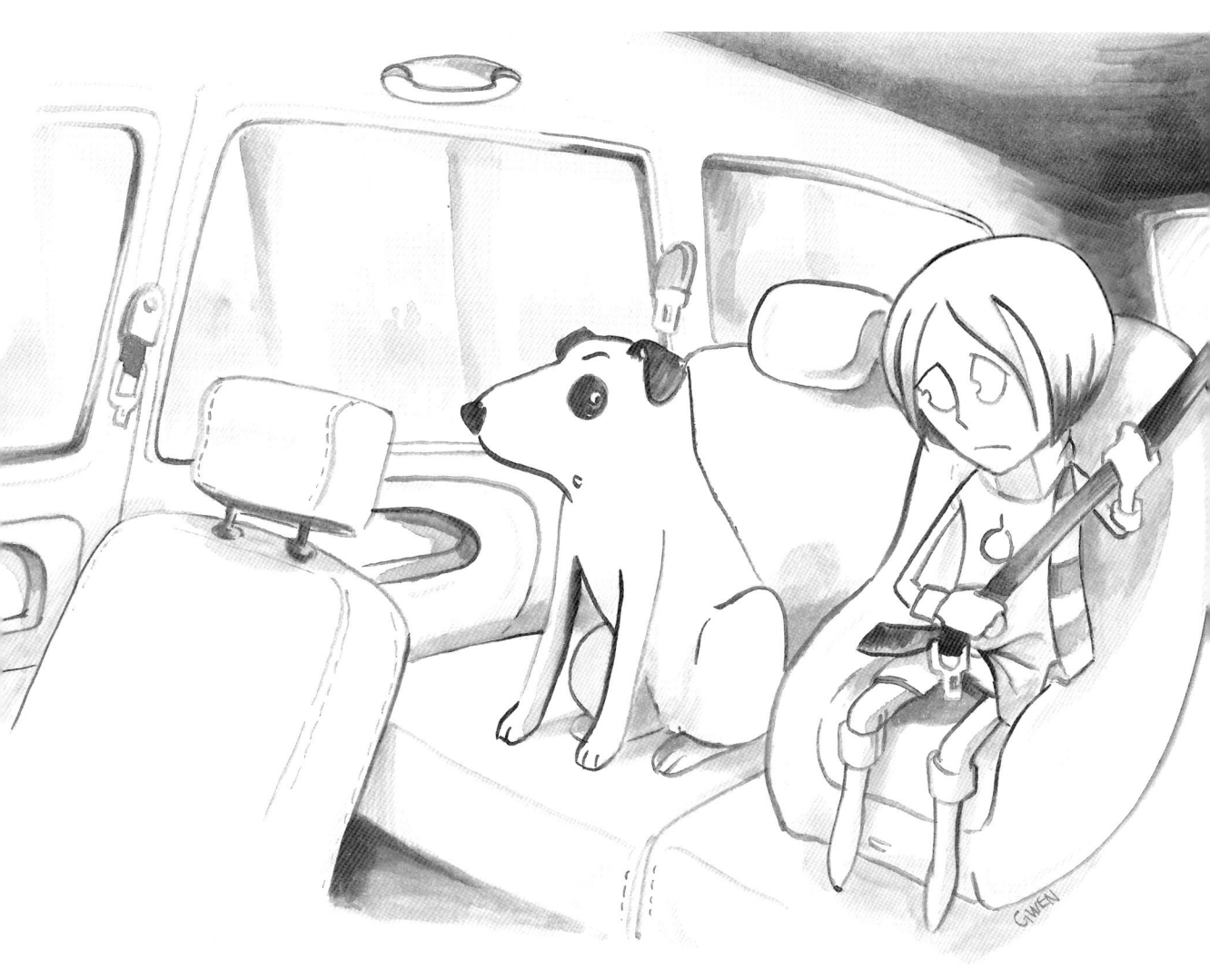

"Sometimes the radiation therapy might be hard on Dad," Mum added. "He might feel very tired. He might have cramps in his stomach, or diarrhoea. He might feel uncomfortable and not want to play."

"Today, cancer is just making me very tired," said Dad. Ella didn't want to talk about it anymore. The forest didn't feel very magical today.
"Can we go home now?" she asked.

Ella didn't say very much on the walk back to the car. She felt guilty for making such a fuss when the walk was cut short. She had lots of questions but was too afraid to ask. Dad said hopefully the cancer would go away, she thought. Does that mean he might be sick forever? What about the hospital? Would he have to stay at the hospital overnight?

Her mind kept whirring all the way home. What if the cancer doesn't go away? Ella wondered.

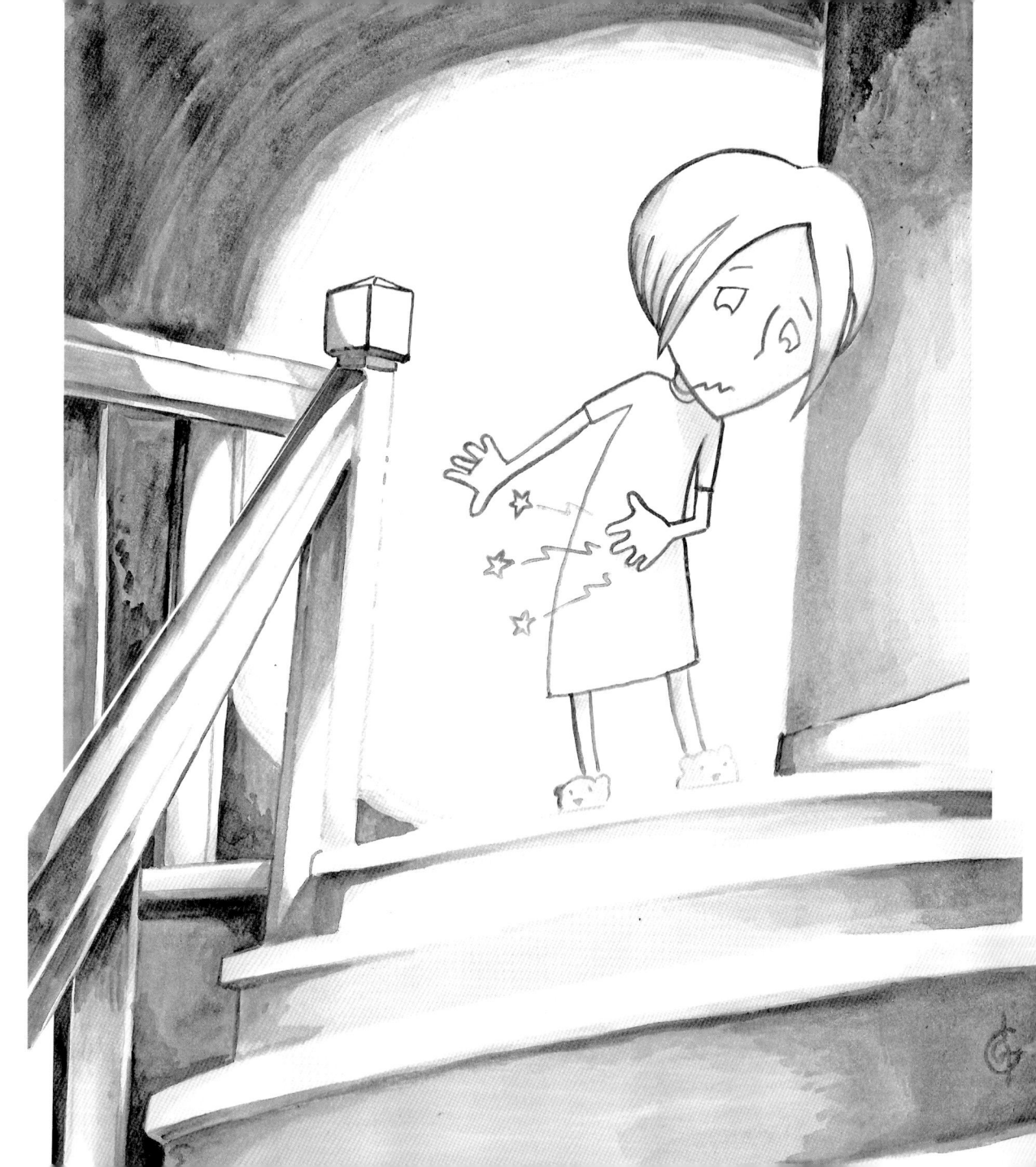

After Ella changed clothes and washed up, her stomach began to feel sore. She remembered what Mum had said, that Dad might have a sore stomach at times. Oh no, Ella thought. Maybe I have cancer too.

Dad usually made a roast after their walk, but no one was very hungry, so he made cheese on toast instead. After they had eaten, the family snuggled up on the couch together. Mum chose a movie to watch, but Ella couldn't concentrate. All she could think about was Dad having cancer. The more Ella thought about cancer, the more anxious she felt. The more anxious she became, the more her stomach ached.

"Mum?" she whispered. "Dad? My stomach really hurts and I feel really tired. Do I have cancer too?"

Mum and Dad exchanged a glance and put their arms around Ella, who was sitting in between them.

"Remember, honey, you can't catch cancer like you can catch a cold," said Mum. "But worrying can make your stomach hurt. Do you think you might be feeling this way because you're worried about Dad?"

Ella thought that Mum was probably right and snuggled into her parents as she tried to settle down to watch the movie.

Chapter Five

When Ella woke up the next morning, the first thing she thought about was Dad having cancer. She felt sad, and still a bit confused. She stayed in bed a little longer than usual, hugging her favourite cuddly toy until Mum called her down for breakfast.

Ella plodded downstairs to the kitchen and sat at the table. Mum placed a fancy glass in front of her, filled with layers of fruit and yoghurt and homemade granola. It looked just like an ice cream sundae. What a treat! She even had a long, fancy spoon to eat it with. Ella forgot her worries. Her stomach didn't ache at all.

After breakfast, Mum walked Ella to the school bus stop. They always called for Ella's best friend, May, on the way.

"Have a great day!" called Mum, waving as the children climbed on the bus. It was a special week at school. All the lessons were going to be dedicated to science, health, and physical activity. The week would be full of different and exciting activities. That morning they were having a health class with Mr Brown – one of Ella's favourite teachers.

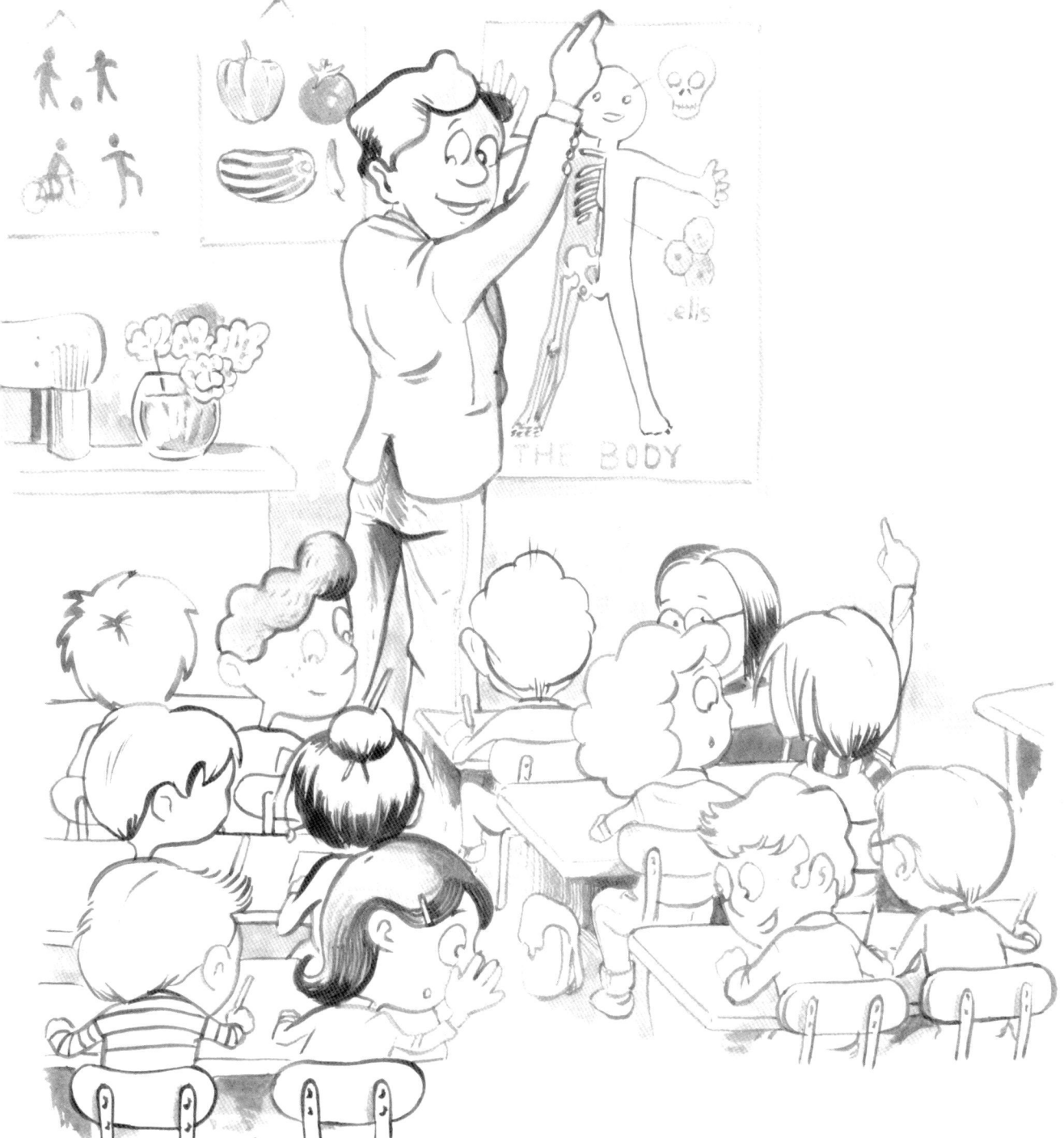

As the children settled into their seats, Mr Brown pinned a poster up at the front of the class. It showed a large image of the human body. Down the side were lots of smaller images – including one image of a cell.

"Our bodies are made up of lots of tiny parts called cells," explained Mr Brown. "The cells in our body are incredibly small. Nowhere near this big," he said, pointing at the image on the poster. "So small, in fact, that you need a microscope to see them clearly."

"What's a microscope?" asked Eric.

"A microscope is just like a magnifying glass, but much stronger. A microscope makes objects appear larger than they actually are."
All of the children nodded.

"Our bodies are made up of lots of tiny cells, and every cell has a special job to do. Some cells help our bones grow strong. Some cells help our brains to think. Other cells help us to feel better after a cold or the flu. And all of our cells work together to keep us healthy." Ella listened to Mr Brown very carefully.

She wondered if he knew anything about cancer. Ella raised her hand.

"What about cancer?" she asked. "What happens to someone's cells if they have cancer?"

Mr Brown explained that cancer occurs when cells become unhealthy. "Cancer is essentially lots of unhealthy cells that grow and take up space where the healthy cells are supposed to be," he said. "But it's not always easy to know when cells have stopped working properly."

"And because our cells are so tiny, and on the inside of our bodies, we can't see what's going on," said Ella confidently.

"That's correct," responded Mr Brown. "A person with cancer doesn't always feel unwell right away. It might take some time to realise something is wrong."

"So how can we keep our cells healthy?" asked Malik.
"What can we do to be sure that we don't get cancer?"

Mr Brown took a moment to think about his answer. "Most often, cancer is found in much older people," he explained. "As people age, their bodies don't work as well as they did when they were younger. But people of all ages can get cancer," he said. "There are certain things you can do to help prevent illness, including cancer." He pointed to some posters he'd put up around the room. One poster showed different types of fruits, vegetables, nuts, and grains. Another poster showed lots of different types of physical activity. "Any ideas what those things might be?" he asked the class.

"You can eat healthy food," said Samira.

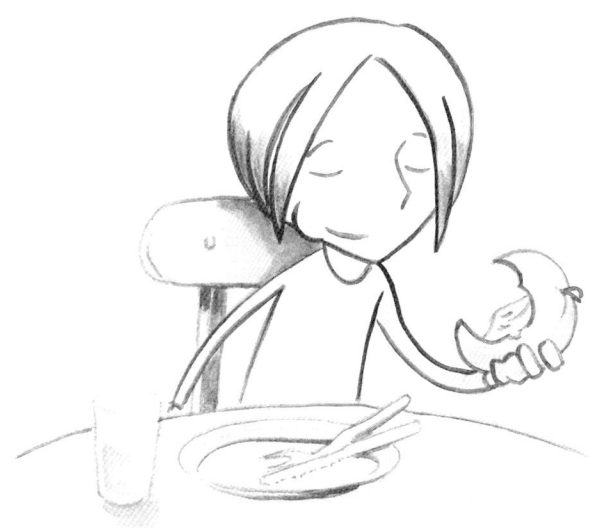

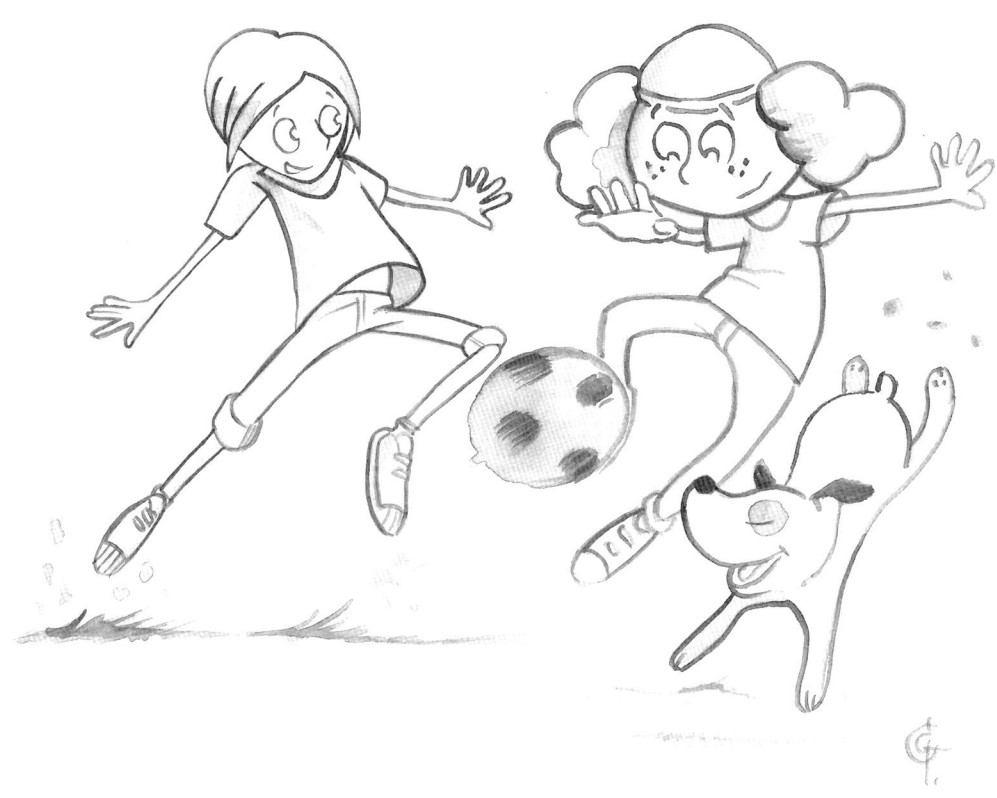

"And get plenty of exercise," added Robbie.

"That's right," said Mr Brown. "And if you feel unwell you can tell your parents and visit the doctor. Remember, it's very important to treat your bodies well," he continued. "For example, it's important not to eat too much sugar and, when you're older, not to smoke cigarettes."

They had talked so much about health and the human body that it was time for a break outside in the fresh air. May waited at the classroom door for Ella. She was curious about Ella's questions.

"Kind of interesting what Mr Brown was saying about our cells," said May.

Ella was quiet.

"Why were you asking all those questions about cancer?" May asked.

Ella stared at the ground as they walked over to sit on the school wall. "My Dad…," Ella started, almost whispering. Even though May was her best friend, it was hard to say it out loud. "My Dad has cancer."

May wasn't sure how to respond. She could tell that Ella was upset. "So, that's why you asked Mr Brown all those questions?" she said.

Ella nodded but stayed very quiet.

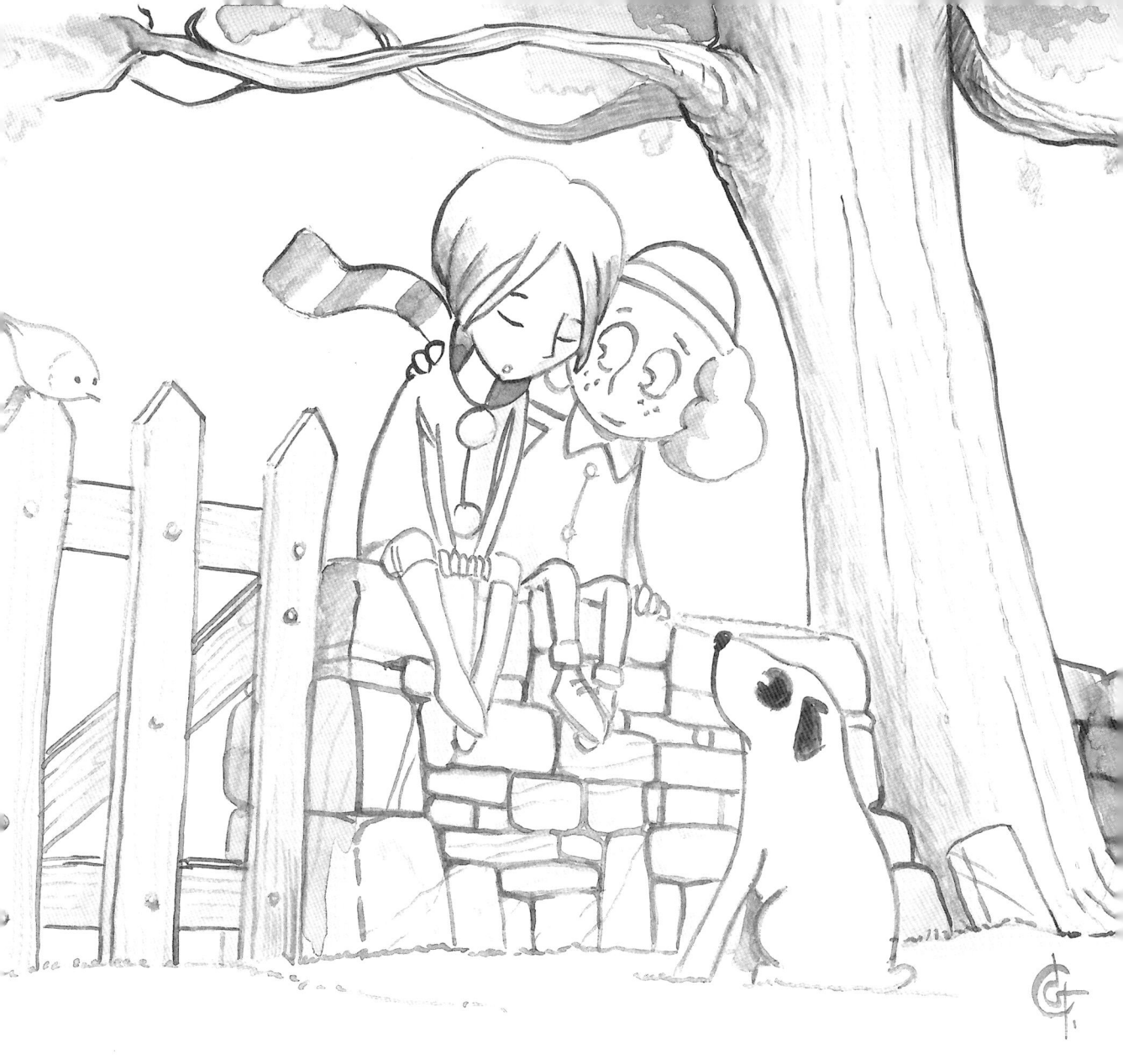

"Does that mean your Dad's cells aren't working the way they're supposed to and he's sick?" asked May.

Ella nodded just as the school bell rang.
May held Ella's hand as they walked back to class.

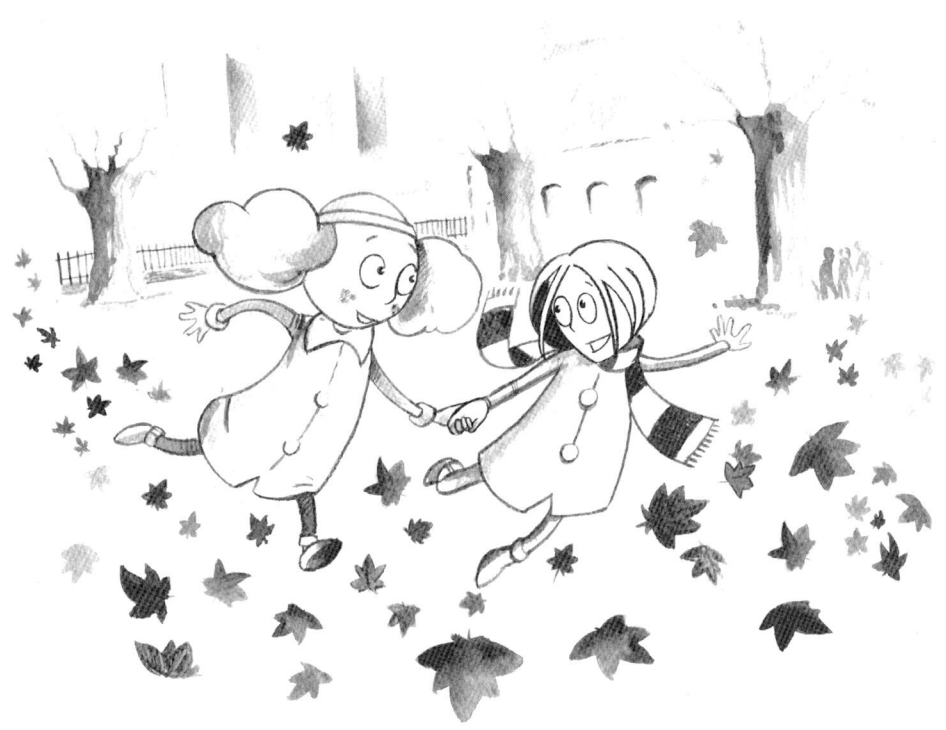

Chapter Six

As usual after school, Ella and May took the school bus back to May's house. On the way, they tried to understand a little bit more about cancer. May asked lots of questions, and Ella tried to explain the best she could. Ella knew that anyone could get cancer. She knew you couldn't catch cancer like you could catch a cold. She knew that cancer occurs when unhealthy cells begin to grow and take up too much space.

The thing that Ella just couldn't understand was how Dad got cancer in the first place.

"It's weird," said Ella. "Dad always eats lots of fruits and vegetables. He always goes jogging with Jasper. Every Sunday we go for a long walk to get exercise. He doesn't smoke cigarettes. Dad does all the things he should do to stay healthy. So, why does he have cancer?"

May didn't have an answer. They decided Ella needed to ask her Dad some more questions.

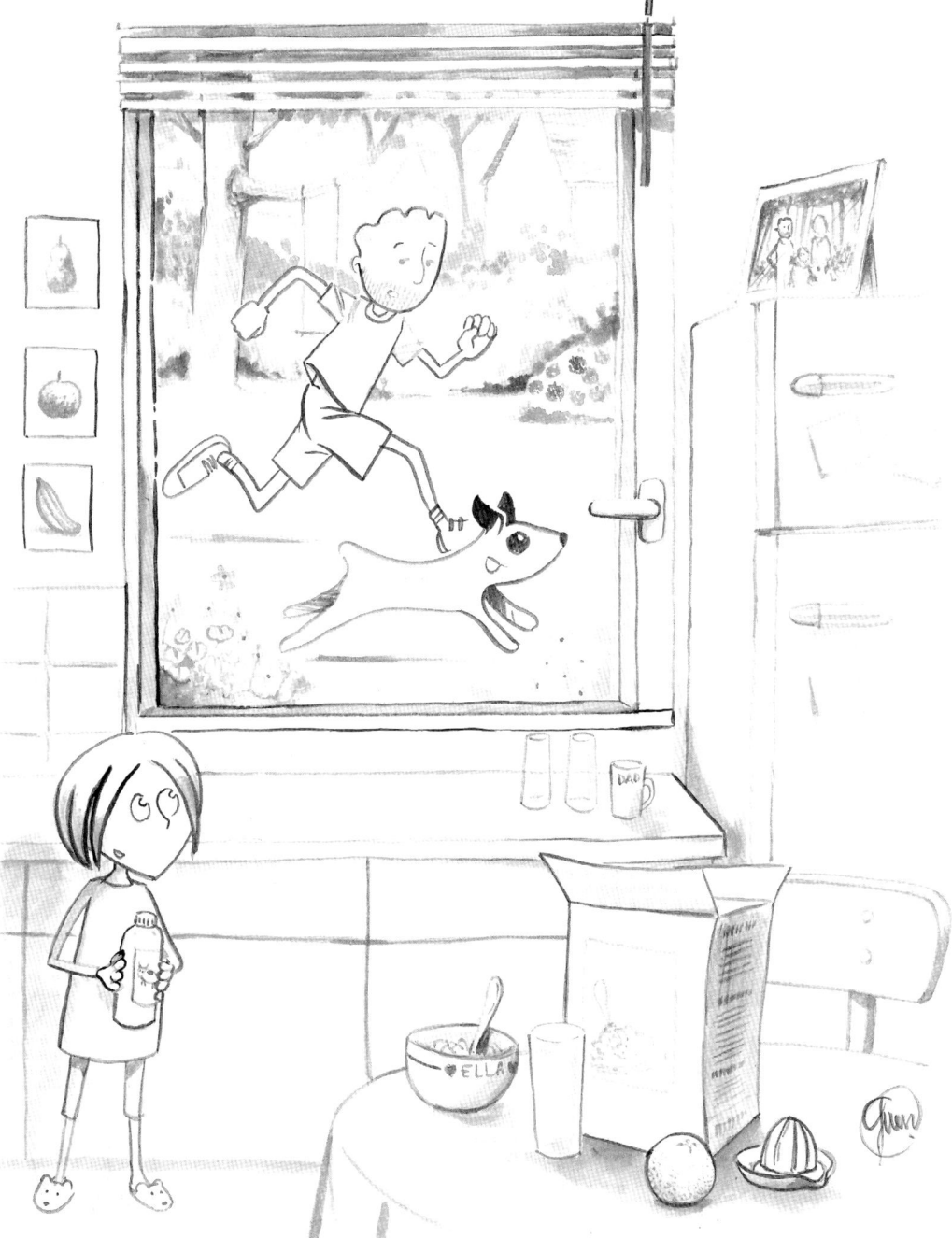

"How was school?" asked Dad when he picked Ella up from May's house a little while later.

"It was pretty good," replied Ella. "It's science, health, and physical activity week. Today we learned about the human body with Mr Brown. He taught us all about cells."

"How interesting," said Dad. "What did you learn?"

"We learned that it's important to eat healthy food and to exercise, but I already knew that," said Ella. "And we learned that our body is made of cells, and that every cell has a special job to do, and that all our cells work together to keep us healthy."

"That's correct," said Dad.

When they got home, Ella helped Dad to prepare dinner. While she was washing the vegetables, Ella thought about the healthy food they were preparing. "Dad, you're always so healthy. How did you get cancer in the first place?"

"That's an excellent question," said Dad. "The type of cancer I have is caused by genetics."

Ella looked confused. Genetics was another word she didn't understand.

"Even though I have healthy habits," explained Dad, "my genetic code caused me to get cancer."

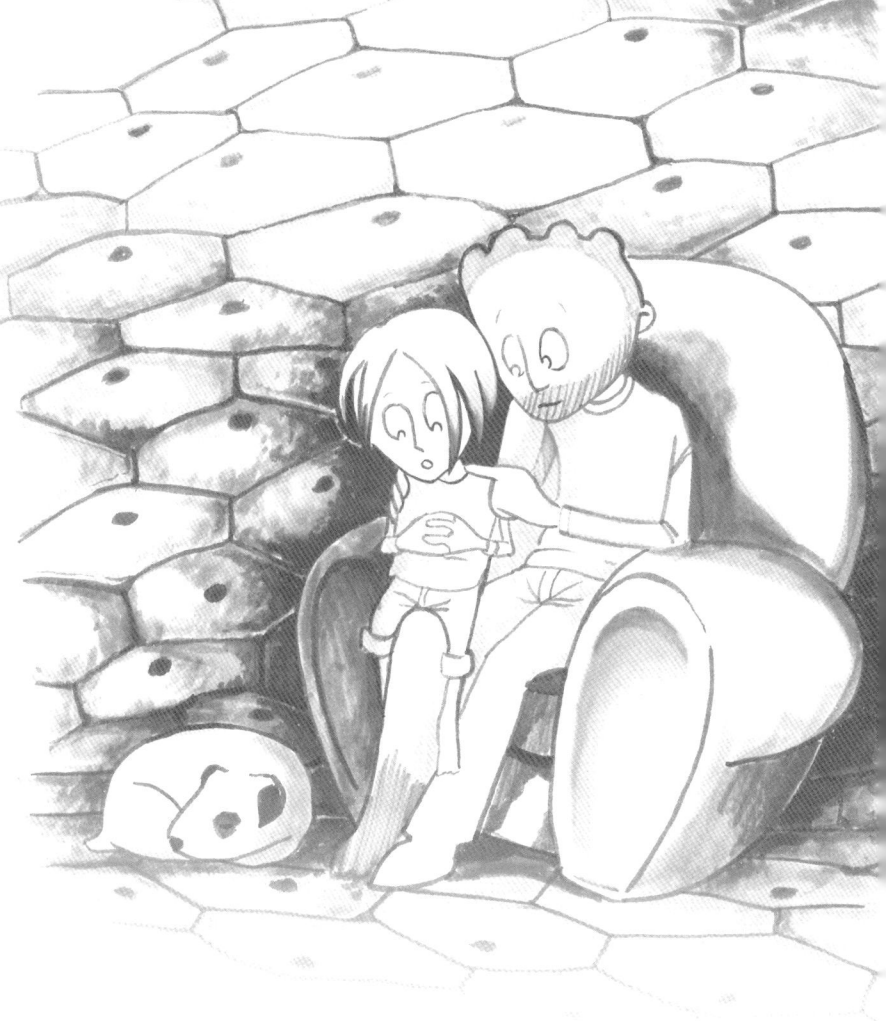

"I don't understand," said Ella, frustrated. "What does that mean?" Dad pulled Ella up onto his knee and tried harder to explain.

"Mr Brown was right," Dad said. "The cells in our bodies are very important. They need to work properly to protect us from diseases like cancer, and we can help them do that by being healthy," Dad said. "But sometimes, because of our genetic code, the cells in our bodies change and grow and multiply and become unhealthy anyway. Cancer can grow simply because of our DNA. And our DNA cannot be changed, no matter what we do."

"What's DNA?" asked Ella, feeling even more confused.

"This might be a little difficult to understand," said Dad. "Remember the building blocks that we always play with?"

Ella nodded.

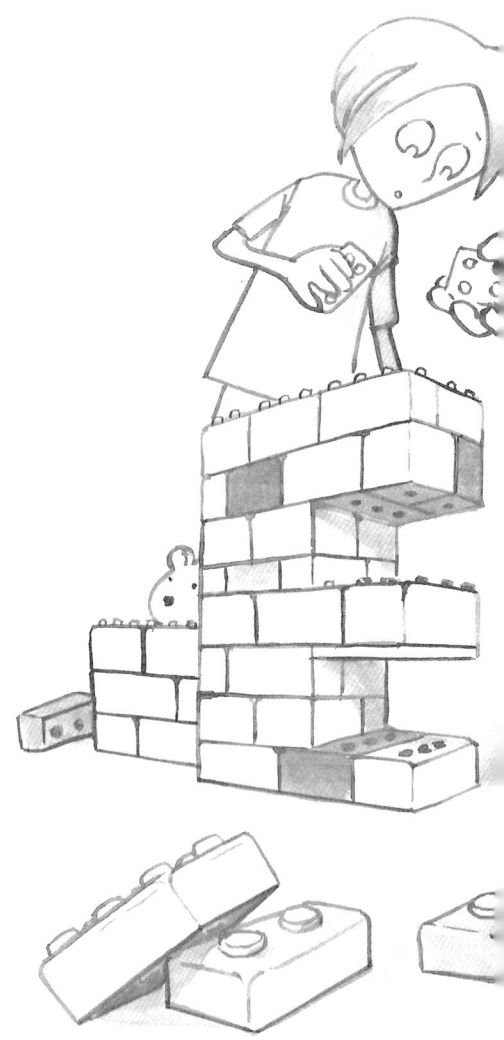

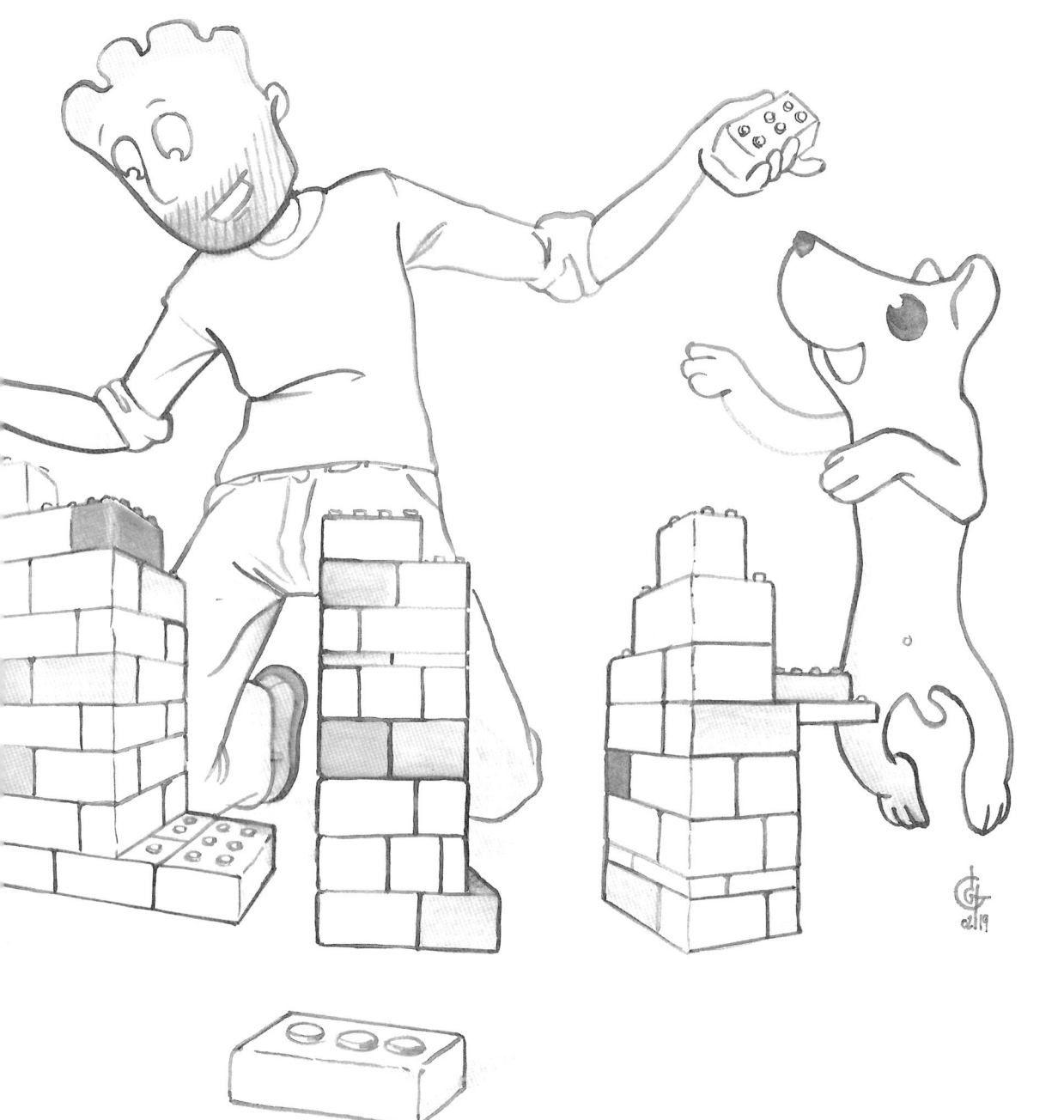

"Our DNA is kind of like our building blocks. When all the blocks fit together just right, we can build a tall, straight tower. But if even one of the blocks doesn't fit because it's the wrong shape or the wrong size, then the tower we build will be lopsided. It might topple over."

"That's right!" said Ella, suddenly understanding.
"All the blocks have to fit together."

"Exactly," said Dad. "I have a wonky block in my DNA that caused me to have cancer, just like the wonky building blocks cause a lopsided tower. If all the building blocks of our DNA fit precisely together, we can stay healthy, but sometimes when they don't quite fit together, we can become unwell, no matter how much broccoli we eat."

Thanks to Mum and Dad and Mr Brown, things were beginning to make a little more sense to Ella. She was beginning to understand a bit more about cancer.

"Dad," said Ella. "I've forgotten whether you told me. Did the doctor give you any medicine to make the cancer go away?"

"Don't worry about forgetting," said Dad. "There's a lot of information to take in. And that's an important question. You can ask me as many questions as you want. Even if you've asked them many times before."

Ella began setting the table for dinner.

"I'm not taking any medication right now," Dad said. "But do you remember I said that I'm going to have some treatment called radiation therapy?"

"Oh yes," said Ella. "The doctor is going to zap the cancer cells with a laser beam. But won't the laser beam hurt you?"

"The most important thing is for the radiation to zap away all the cancer cells. It won't hurt, but I might feel unwell after the treatment. Do you remember what Mum said yesterday?"

"Yes," replied Ella. "Mum said you might have a sore stomach, or have diarrhoea, or be too tired to play."

"That's right," said Dad, carrying the water jug to the table. "But even if I'm too tired to pick you up from May's after school, or I'm too tired to play, or to go for our Sunday walk, remember that I love you very much."

The clock in the kitchen said 5 p.m., which meant that Mum would be home any minute. Ella understood a lot more, but she still had one more question to ask Dad, and it was the biggest and scariest question of all.

Chapter Seven

"How was school today?" asked Mum when the family sat down to dinner. Ella was quiet. She was thinking about the big, scary question she wanted to ask Dad.

"Ella had a great day at school," said Dad. "It's science week, and Mr Brown taught the class all about the human body and cells."

"Science week," said Mum, in between bites. "How fun!"

"And this afternoon we had a chat about genetics and my cancer treatment," said Dad.

Ella was pushing her food around her plate with her fork. She tried to ask Dad the question, but it felt like there was a lump in her throat – no sound came out.

"Ella?" asked Mum. "Are you okay, sweetheart? Is there something you're trying to say?"

Ella tried to ask the question again. She'd managed to get rid of the lump in her throat, but her question came out as a whisper. "Dad," she said. "What will happen if the laser doesn't zap away all the cancer cells? What if the cancer doesn't go away? Will you…" Ella's voice trailed off.

"Will I what?" asked Dad, putting down his cutlery and reaching his hand across the table to Ella.

"Will you die?" asked Ella, finally.

This was a big and scary question indeed. Ella felt hot and sweaty. She stared down at Jasper, who was lapping up water from his bowl, and waited for an answer. Her heart was beating loudly in her ears.

Dad ducked his head to look Ella in the eye and squeezed her hand. "Just like everyone is born," he said, "everyone will also die."

Ella nodded her head. She remembered talking about this once before.

"And yes," said Dad, "some people do die of cancer."

Ella gulped. She felt sick.

"But don't worry," he said. "I went to see the doctor as soon as I was feeling unwell, so she found the cancer at a very early stage. And next week I'll start the radiation therapy. I'm getting the care that I need to help me live a long and healthy life."

Ella felt relieved. She tried to eat some of her dinner, but Mum said it was okay if she wasn't hungry. It had been a long day and Ella was tired.

"I have an idea," said Mum. "Let's think of some activities we can all do together when Dad is feeling unwell after his treatment."

Ella thought that was a great idea. "We could have an indoor picnic!" suggested Ella. "We can lay the picnic blanket on the floor and if Dad is feeling poorly he can lie on the couch but still join in."
Mum and Dad thought that was a wonderful idea.

"Perhaps you can read to Dad if he's tired," suggested Mum. Dad and Ella thought that was a great idea.

"As long as I get to choose the book," said Ella. "Dad's history books are so boring," she added with a giggle. Mum and Dad were smiling.

Soon it was time for bed and Ella went upstairs to brush her teeth. Mum and Dad came up to read her a story and say goodnight. Dad tucked Ella under the covers next to all her cuddly toys. The solar system stickers on Ella's bedroom ceiling glowed above her.

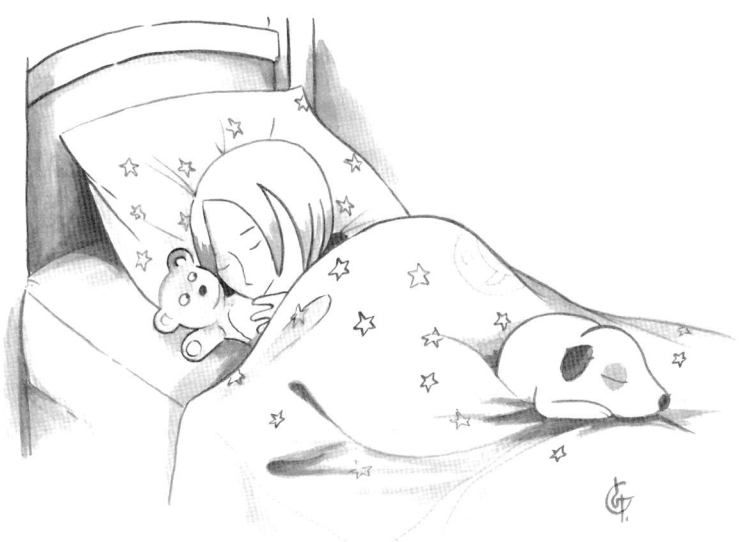

Ella still felt a bit worried, but at least she knew what cancer was and that Dad was starting treatment next week. She understood that Dad would feel poorly after the treatment and was glad they had thought of some activities that everyone could enjoy, even if Dad was unwell. She still wished that Dad didn't have cancer, but at least now she understood that lots of people get cancer and that she wasn't alone. Mum and Dad kissed Ella goodnight.

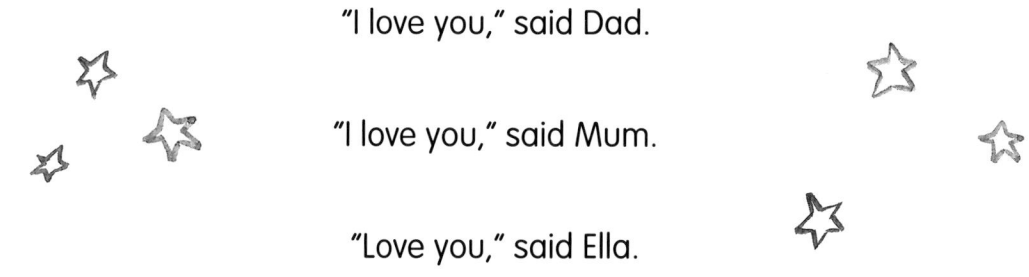

"I love you," said Dad.

"I love you," said Mum.

"Love you," said Ella.

Mum and Dad left the bedroom door ajar so Ella could see Jasper lying on the floor in the hallway. It wasn't long before Ella was fast asleep and dreaming of all the fun she would have with Mum and Dad and Jasper.

The End

Questions and Answers

What is cancer?

Cancer is a disease caused by unhealthy and abnormal cells that continue to grow and multiply without stopping. Cancer can start in any cell, anywhere in the human body, and grow from there. Sometimes, when the cancerous cells grow really quickly and in large amounts, they form a tumour.

What is a tumour?

A tumour is a group of unhealthy and abnormal cells that continue to grow and multiply without stopping. With some types of tumours (malignant tumours),
cells can break off, move to another part of the body, and form another tumour there. With other types of tumours (benign tumours), this does not happen.

What causes cancer?

All cancer is caused by changes in a person's DNA. Strands of DNA are the building blocks of the human body. For some people, changes in DNA that cause cancer are always present, no matter how healthy they are otherwise. For other people, changes in DNA that cause cancer happen because of different things they are exposed to, like tobacco smoke, alcohol, or ultraviolet radiation from the sun.

Will I get cancer if someone I know has cancer?

It's important to remember that you can't catch cancer like you can catch a cold. You can't catch cancer by being close to someone who has cancer, or by hugging them if they feel unwell. However, some types of cancer affect more than one person in a family because family members share some of the same DNA. Some family members have a higher risk of getting cancer because of their shared DNA.

What can I do to prevent cancer?

It's very important to live a healthy lifestyle: for example, to eat fresh fruits and vegetables, not eat too much sugar, and get plenty of exercise. When you are older, it's also important to only drink alcohol in moderation and not to smoke cigarettes. If you're feeling unwell, it's important to talk to someone you trust, like a family member, a teacher, or your family doctor.

Is there a cure for cancer?

There is no known cure for cancer, but there are many different types of treatment for cancer, depending on the type of cancer someone has and how far the cancer has developed.

How is cancer treated?

Most types of cancer can be treated with chemotherapy, radiation therapy, or surgery. In chemotherapy, a person who has cancer will take strong medication to kill the cancer cells. In radiation therapy, cancer cells and tumours will be "zapped" by a beam of radiation. Surgery can be used to remove a cancerous tumour from the body. Some people with cancer will only have one type of treatment, but most people with cancer will have a mixture of treatments for the best possible result.

Other types of treatment include immunotherapy and hormone therapy. Immunotherapy helps a person's immune system fight cancer. Hormone therapy slows down and stops the growth of tumours in some types of cancer. Sometimes a person with cancer will need to be given stem cells or bone marrow cells to help their blood stay healthy.

Does the treatment for cancer hurt?

Some types of cancer treatment do hurt. For example, if someone has surgery to remove a tumour, they will feel sore afterwards. Cancer treatment can make someone feel very ill and tired, or sick to their stomach. Sometimes, if a person has chemotherapy, their hair will fall out. They might have a cough, or a fever, or a headache and be unable to play. A person being treated for cancer will need lots of time to rest to help them feel better.

Will cancer come back after it is treated?

Some forms of cancer will not come back after they have been treated, but some forms of cancer will come back. That's why most people with cancer need more than one type of treatment, and that's why it's important to find cancer at a very early stage when it is only just beginning to grow. All forms of treatment are most effective when cancer is at a very early stage, and that's when cancer is less likely to come back after it is treated.

What is IARC?

IARC is the International Agency for Research on Cancer – the specialized cancer agency of the World Health Organization. IARC is located in Lyon, France, and was established in May 1965. IARC's mission is: Cancer research for cancer prevention.
You can learn more about IARC from the agency's website, which is available in both English and French: **www.iarc.fr**.

Where do the proceeds from the sale of this book go?

100% of the proceeds from the sale of this book go to the education and training of cancer researchers worldwide. This is a core part of IARC's mission, which is achieved through fellowships, courses, and publications.

About the author

Dr Tricia L. Larose is from Sudbury, a city in Ontario, Canada. She holds a PhD in Medicine from the Norwegian University of Science and Technology. Her work is supported by the Research Council of Norway (grant number 267776/H10). During her tenure as a postdoctoral scientist at the International Agency for Research on Cancer (IARC), Dr Larose worked in the Genetic Epidemiology Group in the Section of Genetics.

About the illustrator

Gwen Le Rest is an illustrator and sculptor. His illustrations for this book were inspired by his five children. He sometimes publishes work under the pseudonym Géhélère (GLR). His artist's studio is located in Locunolé, a village in Brittany in north-western France.

About the editor

Beth Cox is based in Wiltshire in the United Kingdom. She has worked with children's books for all ages – from birth to young adult (YA) – since 2003. She is a specialist in inclusion and diversity and is the co-founder of Inclusive Minds®.